Naturopathy for Beginners

Evolve to the Alternate Form of Naturopathic Medicine for a Healthier, More Natural You

By Ursula Jamieson

Published in Canada

© Copyright 2015 – Ursula Jamieson

ISBN-13: 978-1511440424
ISBN-10: 1511440422

ALL RIGHTS RESERVED. No part of this publication may be reproduced or transmitted in any form whatsoever, electronic, or mechanical, including photocopying, recording, or by any informational storage or retrieval system without express written, dated and signed permission from the author.

Table of Contents

Introduction 1
Chapter 1: The Philosophy Behind Naturopathy 3
Chapter 2: The Benefits of Naturopathy 8
Chapter 3: Naturopathic Treatments 11
    Yoga 11
    Acupuncture 14
    Color Therapy 16
    Reiki 18
    Homeopathy 20
    Ayurvedic Medicine 22
    Aromatherapy 24
Chapter 4: How to Use Naturopathy in Your Daily Life 25
Conclusion 29

Introduction

In recent years, people have been increasingly concerned about their health and natural treatments, and the promising discipline of naturopathy has consequently and quickly gained ground. While only a few years ago everybody would rush to the doctor at the first signs of any disease, now the number of people who believe in the powers of modern medicine have decreased considerably. Sometimes, the chemicals that found in medicinescan be more damaging than helpful tothe body. Moreover, most people have already developed an immunity to a large number of antibiotics or drugs used in modern medicines.

Naturopathyhas proven itself to be as effective, but not as damaging, as any other modern treatment. It is a type of alternative medicine that does not use modern drugs and chemicals. Practitioners of naturopathic medicine believe that the body has the power to heal itself without the intervention of chemicals. The body already has the necessary instruments to become healthy;it just needs to know how to use them.

Naturopathy includes a wide variety of natural treatments and uses a holistic approach to any medical affliction. This type of alternative medicine combines authentic knowledge with the discoveries of modern science and brings a new way of treating the body without risking long term injury. The roots of naturopathy go back thousands of years, and since ancient times, people have used the benefits of nature to maintain their health.

The procedures are meant to be as minimally invasive as possible. Surgery and modern medicine are recommended only in extreme cases.Otherwise the body's energy, together with natural ingredients, is all that is needed to heal almost any disease. Additionally, naturopathy emphasizes the importance of careful prevention, rather than desperate treatment.

This book provides insight into the most common practices of naturopathy and how they are used to treat different afflictions. Many of the natural remedies that are used can be prepared in yourown home,allowing you to find asolutionwithout common medicines to problems that have bothered you for years.

Naturopathy uses meditation, fragrances, physical activity, and acupuncture, apart from other prepared remedies. They work together to reach the supreme goal of any person: a perfect balance between body, mind, and spirit.

Chapter 1: The Philosophy Behind Naturopathy

Some people call naturopathy "the science of living" and they lead their lives under the main principles of this science. They do this because naturopathy is not meant to only provide alternative treatment to ailments; it is meant to combine the healing of the body, mind, and spirit. Proponents of naturopathy say that you cannot be healthy if one of these elements is impure. Therefore, you need to be in complete harmony with yourself and with the nature around you to live your life to itsmaximum potential.

Modern medicine frequently ignores the energy of our body. However, this energy is our main ally when we want to change our life and become healthy and happy. Those who adopt naturopathy as a way of living do not simply stop taking modern medicines, but they change everything about their life. Their food, their perspectives about the surrounding environment and their dedications to leading a complete and healthy life are altered. When one removes the negative elements that surround them, there is more space to embrace positive energy.

Mental and spiritual power is a very important part of the healing process for any injury or illness. The body is also influenced not only by external factors life food and environment, but also by negative thoughts and energies from within. Very often when a person receives bad news or is upset that individual can start to feel bad physicallybecause can emotions have a terrible impact on our health. To ensure perfect functioning of the body, it is important to limit negative thoughts and to learn how to control emotions. Whenevera person becomes frustrated, very often by events beyond control, that person is damaging the body and the spirit. Conversely when one isin complete control ofthe mind, health starts to improve noticeably.

This concept of emotions affecting one's health is one that healers have always known, and now one that modern medicine embraces. If you are happy, your body will heal itself. Very often doctors will use, as last resort, the "Placebo Effect" on patients. Under this practice, doctorsadminister fake medicine and let patients think that they these treatments will help them become healthy. And in fact, most of these patients do become healthy. Very sick patients, with cancer or other terminal illnesses, haverecovered in course of just months using the Placebo Effect. These "magical" recoveriesare proof that, by using positive energy and the power of spirit, people can solve problems that seem impossible to overcome. Unfortunately, people are often so trapped in the superficial world where everything has a material response that they forget that people are much more than flesh and bones.

The body's energy can make people capable of amazing feats. A case that brought naturopathy to the public's attention was a tragic accident in the United Statesseveral years ago. A woman saw her child trapped under a car, and she consequently managed to lift the car – weighing 2,000 pounds, by herself. Scientists said that this was merely the result of an excess of adrenaline, but this only confirms the main idea of naturopathy. We have an amazing power that we simply do not know how to use.

Many people think that naturopathic doctors are health gurus that study ancient books and derive their core knowledge from myths. In reality, they study the same basic sciences as any mainstream doctor, but they choose a different approach,believing prevention is more important than treatment.Naturopathy is not, as mainstream media promotes purposely or inadvertently, just about using herbs and meditation to heal a common cold.

Most of the treatments using naturopathic medicine are at least approved, if not recommended, by modern medicine. The difference between the two is that modern medicine is using ingredients that are processed so intensely that they lose all of their keybenefits, while naturopathic medicine uses those same ingredients in their pure form.

When doctors recommend that a patient rests, avoids processed food and drinks a lot of liquids, without knowing, those doctors are recommending naturopathic treatments. A healthy, balanced way of life is what people need to cure themselves of most illnesses, not several novel medicines. It is more logical to prevent an illness from happening than to treat each one after it arrives. Of course, one can take a pill to get rid of a headache, but that does not find or treat the main cause of pain. This means that the problem will continue to appear until that individual is ultimately addicted to medicines.

There are many types of treatment used in alternative medicine, each one being effective in aiding certain problem areas that people tend to encounter. Meditation, physical activities, and a vegan diet are all part of naturopathy; they all stimulate or repair natural defense systems while maintaining natural chemical balances in the body.

Most people are very reluctant when they first try to employ naturopathy. It seems unbelievable that meditation and plants can heal problems that were too big for modern medicine to tackle. There is one principle that supports the entireideology behind naturopathy: we have all of the weapons we need to fight any disease in ourselves. The body is designed to heal itself,but its natural processes will do this only if it is provided with a suitable environment.

When we chose pills laden with hidden toxins, we stop the natural healing processes,and we disturb the chemical composition of our body. The fact that mortality rates from diseases is increasing annually proves that modern medicine has failed. Ultimately, if these toxic medicines were as effective as they are presented to be, the mortality rates would be decreasing, and we would have fewer sick patients every year. A realistic look at the situation indicates that we need to go back to our roots and to use the resources we have always had.

Chapter 2:
The Benefits of Naturopathy

There are many known benefits of naturopathy, but we are going to list the most common and important ones.

First, naturopathy is the medicine of the soul and spirit. It is not just another type of medicine that will take away your headaches; it can be one of the best actions you take in your life. People who started applying naturopathic principles discovered how, day by day, their life changed. Beyond a healthy blood pressure or pain relief, this new way of life changed their mentality. A different approach to life can lead to improvement every single aspect of it that was bothering you or that was creating discomfort. It canalso create peace and tranquility that no other type of medicine or therapy can bring you.

For example many doctors recommend naturopathic treatments for patients who suffer from severe depressionbecause it takes much more than a few pills to heal the spirit.

Additionally naturopathycan stimulate the body's capacity for regeneration by opening the energy flow that is blocked by years of modern aliments and stressful schedules. When you find yourself suddenly enduring pain or migraines it is not because you did not get enough sleep. It is because your body, your mind, and your spirit are not in complete harmony, and you need to bring balance to your life. Once you start applying thenaturopathic science to your life, relationships with others will improve dramatically. A happy person that spreads positive energy will be like a magnet for the people who seek an escape from their own stressful lives.

The third, and perhaps biggest, advantage of naturopathy is that it keeps you away from toxic ingredients found in medicine. Chemicals, even if they are meant to heal you, will always cause an imbalance in the chemical composition of your body and will cause much more bad than good in the long run. Moreover, when you consume a lot of medicines you can develop a high risk of depression and anxiety because many of the drugs inhibit the natural production of endorphinswhich are the hormones that make us happy.

If you are searching for effective remedies for a medical condition, you will be happy to discover out that naturopathy can help to heal most of the diseases that modern medicinecan only provide comfort for. There are certain cases where naturopathic principles have been applied successfully in difficult situations, including terminal patients or individuals with dangerous tumors. However, most peopleuse naturopathy to seek solutions to more simple problems, such as afflictions of the digestive tract or insomnia. Many simple treatments including homeopathy or herbal infusions can heal these medical problems withoutthe use of any chemicals.

Finally, many skin diseases can be healed through acupuncture or the use of natural lotions. The lotions that are often prescribed by doctorsare basedin natural ingredients. However these lotions lose their healing properties in the production process, and the active ingredients become an insignificant part of the final product. If you want a beauty treatment, it is always more effective to replace modern cosmetics with natural alternatives. These will not only make you look younger, but it will also preserve your health and give your skin the natural supplements that it needs to shine.

In sum there are very few medical afflictions that naturopathy cannot heal. Except for those cases that require surgical intervention, our body contains all of the resources that it needs to heal and function properly. All we need to do is to learn how to use them and to live our life to our full capacity.

Chapter 3: Naturopathic Treatments

Yoga

Yoga is one of the best ways to gain control over your body, mind and spirit. It is, surprisingly, the solution for many problems that we encounter in our day-to-day life. Some people consider it an art, some people practice it as a sport, and some people simply seek the calming effects of the meditation that works in conjunction with the practice. What began as an old, Indian art is now one of the most widely used ways of spiritual healing.

Practicing Yoga works your mind, body and spirit, and it is considered by naturopath practitioners to be the best way to prevent and heal any affliction. One of the most effective methods of gaining mental stability, the meditative part of Yoga has helped many people where traditional medicine did not have any effect. Yoga teachespeople how to be in complete harmony with the world around them by connecting them totheir deepest thoughts. While revealing and directing the body's natural energy, people can discover a new and fascinating world where they are in control of everything. People have little control over what happens to them, but they can have complete control over how they react to it. You cannot make your boss less cranky, but you can change how such person's behavior affects your mood if you are in control of your feelings.

Yoga is a complex science that covers many areas of our mental and physical health. Constant practicecan lead to a more balanced way of life, and often causes a change one's the daily alimentation. Many who practice yoga ultimately becomevegetarians. One of the basic principles of yoga, and naturopathy in general, is that in order to be healthy, it is important to build one's alimentation on natural, unprocessedingredients. Yogis, the people who practice Yoga, usually consider ingesting animal products astaking in negative energy that can bring an imbalance in the body. Even those who do continue to eat animal products believe that the processed, modern alimentation is one of the main causes of mainstream diseases.

"Asanas" are specific Yoga positions that, when combined with concentrated breathing techniques and meditation, can have healing properties that will bring a variety of benefits to the body. Insomnia, depression, indigestion, and muscular painsfrom a low immune system can all be healed and prevented with the most basic positions of Yoga. Mainstream doctors would likely recommend chemical medicines for these symptoms, butthose are reallyunnecessary. Most often, these biological imbalances are simply a sign that we are not living well, that we have a bad diet, or that we are stressing ourselves out with unimportant matters. Whatever ailment we have that is not caused by a chemical imbalance cannot then be solved with excess of chemicals.

One of the important elements of Yoga is the breathing techniques. By simply controlling your inspiration and expiration you can relax yourself, control your pain and aid sleep disorders. There are many different breathing practices, each one of them suitable for a specific Yoga position. In general, any person can benefit from this practice. You can apply it wherever you are, whenever you want.

Acupuncture

Acupuncture has become widely used in the beauty industry. Apart from the health benefits, the public became familiar with acupuncture when scientist discovered the amazing effect this treatment can have on the skin. An increasing number of people use this treatment to keep their skin young and smooth.

Acupuncture uses a holistic approach for thehealing ofafflictions that are common in modern times. The practice originated in ancient China, and it is now used worldwide as an alternative to modern medicine. The ideology behind acupuncture highlights twelve meridian channels and two central channels that send energy through the body. When one of these channels has a blockage, the rivers of energycannot flow normally, and disturbances in the normal functioning of the body result.This energy is called"Chi" by the practitioners of acupuncture, and its flow is used to alienate pain, to reduce stress or tension and to rejuvenate damaged skin.

The acupuncture process consists of the application of small needles under the skin at key points. Thistreatment restores the balance of energy, and it encourages your body to use its healing power in needed areas. People who could not be diagnosed by a mainstream physicianfound their answers from acupuncture specialists. Energy channels are not accepted as real by the modern medicine. However, an acupuncture specialist will know how to discover and restore the imbalance that is causing your symptoms. One who suffers from insomnia and takes medication for years without success can find a relief after only a few sessions of acupuncture. Even if the application of the needles can be frightening at the first sight, there is no pain and no discomfort.

There are variations to acupuncture where the doctor applies heat or electrical stimulation atcertain points. The electrical stimulation is often used for facial treatments and now it represents one of the most effective treatments for wrinkles and scars. The stimulation of the tissue using electricity encourages the skin to produce collagen, which is the protein that gives elasticity to the skin.

Acupuncture treatment is also used worldwide for the treatment of muscular pain. Introducing the needle at a specific point of the muscle can release tension, and it can alienate the pain almost instantly. Chemical lotions or pills will only treat the symptom, but it will not treat the cause. Conversely, acupuncture will treat the causes and will also prevent future diseases.

Modern medicine has come to accept acupuncture as a legitimate medical practice, and now there are physicians that are being trained in this field. However, it is a treatmentthat has been used for thousands of years, and it is one of the most effective practices from alternative medicine.

Color Therapy

For people who are ready to find alternative solutions fortheir problems, color therapy has proven to be a useful alternative medicine, especially for children. Many people observed, for years, how a certain color used for the walls of the bedroom can induce better sleep. However, complete color therapy has been developed only recently.

Color therapy is one of the easiest ways to prevent afflictions that would otherwise require medical attention. From sleep problems to digestive ailments, the simple effect of a certain color can influence your spirit and your body. Psychologists discovered how chromotherapy is effective, especially for children with autism or Attention Deficit Hyperactivity Disorder, or as a form of cognitive therapy. Chromotherapists say that by using different colors we can actually balance the energy levels of our body, and we can compensate for what we lack. Scientistshave researched the topic and they have discovered how viewing some colors can actually trigger the release of certain hormones in our brain, changing our mood and alienating pain.

Using colors to influence the mood is has come to be used widely in interior design. Designers realized the impact that a color can have on people and how a specific wall color can make the difference between a normal kitchen, and one thatelevates your appetite.

Restaurants, bars, and stores all use the power of colors to trigger feelings and emotions and to influence the clients. Very often, you can notice how a certain color instantly makes you feel happy or sad.

Color therapy is extremely accessible to all people, and you do not need any previous training or complex knowledge to apply it. You simply need to inform yourself about the effect of different colors, and with that information, you can improve your daily life.

Colors do not only have aneffecton our moods, but also our physical selves. Blood pressures can be increased or decreased with the help of the colors red and blue. Digestion can be improved by using the color green in the areas we eat, and we can have a relaxing night's rest if our bedroom is painted in dark colorssuch as burgundy or brown.

Photobiology, the scientific study of different types of lights and color on living organisms,was developed following the appearance of color therapy. Even if modern science does not completely accept thecorrelation between colors and medical treatment, some scientists do admit that it seems to create a positive response in patients that are exposed to different types of lights.

Reiki

We, as human beings, are made up of much more than flesh and bones. We possess an internal energy and force that only naturopaths focus on. Even if modern medicine pretends to have answers to our questions, this is not the truth. Modern medicine is not the answer, but rather, it is just a way of treating the symptoms. When we are sick, we are damaged at a more profound level, in the core of our spirit.

Reiki is an old practice that was recently resurrected by people who believe that we contain the power to heal ourselves. The Reiki ideology focuses on the energetic points of our body called "chakras." These points are localized around our endocrine glands and together they create the invisible, energetic field of our body.We can receive and give energy to all living things around us, from plants to human beings. Reiki practitioners believe that when one of these points is damaged or something stops the flow of energy, we are affected onboth a mental and a physical plane.

Similarly, each person has the internal power to heal through this energy and to heal others. However, most of thepeople do not use this capacity, and they lose it somewhere between childhood and adulthood. The Reiki instructors have maintained or regained this capability, and they teach other people how to use their internal energy to help others.

By opening each chakra and teaching you how to direct your energy, you can send positive vibes through your palms.

People who decide to practice Reiki also vow to change their life in a positive manner. They avoid negative thoughts, learn how to attract positive energy, and understand how to be satisfied with their ownlives. This practice promotes a happy, peaceful life in harmony with everything around you. When somebody gets sick, it is because an energy point is affected by external factors. This means that everytime negative energies exceed the positive energies, there will be negative effects onone's health. A Reiki practitioner can use his own positive energy to heal and to help us regain strength.

There have been provenbenefits for muscular pain, migraines, insomnia, digestive problems, and depression. Some skin diseases can also be healed by using our internal energy. For somebody who leads a stressful, busy life, practicing this type of therapy can be the perfect way to prevent many health problems.

Homeopathy

Homeopathy is a type of holistic medicinebased on the principle that we should treatthe patient, not only the disease. It appeared in the 18th century, and today it is recommended by an increasing number of doctors as an alternative solution.

This type of therapy uses the natural tendency of the body to heal itself. There are two known ways of healing- the similar and the opposed way. Homeopathy uses the similar way,which means that the homeopath doctor will recommend small doses of caffeine that, whenadministered correctly, will have the opposite effect expected.

The medicines that are administrated in homeopathic medicine are not addictive, and they do not damage the body since they are only recommended in very small dosages. They are not meant particularly to heal, but they are utilized to stimulate the body to fight against the disease. There are many homeopathic treatments that are prescribed and recommended by doctors in different branches. The ingredients were, in the beginning,entirely natural, but since homeopathyhas spread all over the world, some remedies are now produced in factories.

The homeopathic treatments are now preferred by many people with allergies or who have developed resistance to modern drugs. One of the main aspects that makes homeopathic treatment so effective is that it is administered and adapted to any patient based on his or her medical history and specific preferences like diet, way of life or stress levels, through a personal medical scheme that is designed by the homeopath doctor. The homeopath doctor will create your personalized scheme of treatment, adapted completely to your needs.

Homeopathy is believed to be, by many people, the ideal alternative to the modern medicine. Instead of focusing only on the symptoms, it preventsmany diseases instead of trying to treat them as they arise. Minimally invasive, the homeopath treatments never change the natural chemical balance of the body, but instead stimulate the natural healing process. When we ingest a medicine that contains toxic ingredients, we are actually changing the chemistry of our body and we are damaging not only its immunity, but also its capacity to fight the diseases long term.

Ayurvedic Medicine

Ayurvedic Medicine is an ancient practice that appeared in India thousands of years ago, and it is based on the Vedic texts, India's sacred books. It is similar to other naturopathic branches, like homeopathy or Chinese herbal medicines. However, distinct from these other natural remedies, it is an entire system based on meditation, Yoga, and a strict diet.

The Ayurvedic lifestyle is based on balance in every aspect of our lives: diet, sleep, sexual relations, emotions, and physical activity. Somebody who decides to try Ayurvedic Medicine will encounter an entire program that needs to be strictly followed in order to obtain the perfect equilibrium between mind, body, and spirit. Most patients start with a careful detoxification, not only physically but also mentally. There are different recommended detoxification diets, from intermittent fasting to herbal drinks.

The practitioners of this discipline believe that it is important to cleanse the body and the mind before we try to heal any damage. Some even maintain extended Water Fasts, from 3 days to several weeks. In this time, they drink only water, and they spend their time practicing light Yoga or other types of meditation. Fasting is a common practice in all religions of the world, and modern medicine has started to accept its benefits.

It is believed that a week of Water Fasting will give your body the opportunity to direct all the energy to healing and not waste time with digestion and absorption. After breaking a fast, most people adopt a diet based solely on fruits and vegetables, reducing or eliminating meat and processed food.

For people who cannot carry out Water Fasts, the practitioners of Ayurvedic Medicine recommend juice fasting to eliminate toxins and to give the body a break. This means that for several days, the patient will only drink natural, fresh juices. People who have tried this said that they do not feel hungry but ratherthey actually stopped having cravings and noticed how they slept less but felt more rested

Aromatherapy

Aromatherapy can be considered an individual practice or a part of Ayurvedic Medicine. It is often combined with fasting and meditation, and it consists of the usage of essential oils or natural extracts as treatment for different conditions.It is true that some fragrances have a positive impact on our general mood, and they can influence our emotional state throughout the day. A delicate scent of vanilla can make us feel relaxed after a busy day and lavender perfume can help us sleep better. However, the effect of fragrances on physical diseases is still a subject of debate.The usage of essential oils has proven to be beneficial for people who suffer from insomnia, digestive problems, anxiety or nausea. By using natural extracts in hot water, you can also relieve the symptoms of the flu or seasonal allergies.

Combined with meditation or Yoga, Aromatherapy has incredible effects onone's mind and spirit. Not only can itrelieve depression, but it can also ameliorate a wide number of psychological afflictions. The practitioners of Ayurvedic Medicine or Reiki always introduce fragrances in their meditation sessions, and they believe it helps the natural flow of energy. In combination with Acupuncture, it can create wonders for pain relief, and patients who were experiencing chronic pain could finally live a normal life. A certain version of aromatherapy is used nowadays in stores and in companies where fragrances are used to make the clients feel comfortable and relaxed.

Chapter 4:
How to Use Naturopathy in Your Daily Life

If you decide to adjust your lifestyle and to use the natural ingredients rather than chemical ones, there are some primary steps you need to take and a certain mindset you need to develop. You do not need to become a Yoga guru or to make sessions of acupuncture every week to practice naturopathy.

There are small adjustments you can make to have a healthier, happier life. Many people apply principles of naturopathy even without realizing it simply by adopting a healthy lifestyle where they prevent instead of treating diseases. A balanced diet, constant physical activity, and a positive attitude are, in the end, naturopathic treatments themselves.

Of course, if you wish to deepen your knowledge about naturopathy, there are always courses that you can take or specialized trainers that you can talk with. Meanwhile, there are some simple remedies that you can apply in your daily life without too much effort.

Insomnia is, maybe, one of the most common sleeping disorders of modern times. Of course, chaotic and stressful lives are the main reasons for this. Instead of pumping yourself with sleeping pills, try some natural remedies that will not damage your body in thelongterm, and they will give you the calm sleep that you wish for. Ashwagandha is an ancient herb that is well-known for its anti-depressant effect. It is used mainly in the Ayurveda Medicine, and it is administered in small dosages before going to sleep, it can put you in a relaxed mood that will eliminate insomnia.

If you want a remedy that does not imply any kind of substance, a short session of Yoga should work as well. Without trying any complicated positions, simply meditate and focus on your breathing for fifteen minutes before going to bed. Your stressful thoughts will disappear immediately, and you will be able to have calm, restful sleep.

To improve your general mood and stimulate your appetite, you can try to apply the principles of color therapy in your home. Paint the walls of your home in colors that will help you manage every aspect of the day. For example, paint the walls in your kitchen or dining room in a dark green to stimulate an appetite and prevent digestive problems. A cozy color in the living room, like beige or light brown,can create an intimate atmosphere and improve the time you spend with your family. For your bedroom, blue will give you a fresh feeling in the morning, while cherry-colored walls will put you in a deep, comfortable sleep. You can also use different objects as colored spots that will boost your mood through the day.

To strengthen your immunities and to prevent seasonal allergies, you can use a homeopathic remedy that is used successfully worldwide. Mix ten teaspoons of honey with three teaspoons of boxthorn and leave the mixture in a closed jar for at least two weeks. A spoonful of this mixture every morning will not only give you energy and improve your digestion, but it will strengthen your immunity, and it will keep you from getting colds in the winter. Moreover, it will keep your appetite under control during the day, and you will not have cravings between meals.

If you experience acne, pimples or frequent breakouts on your skin and you cannot seem to find the cause, a natural ointment made from Mezereummay be effective. Daphne Mezereum is a plant used since ancient times to treat skin diseases or to give a feeling of tranquility to agitated patients. Nowadays, some modern ointments contain this plant but, unfortunately, most of its healing properties are destroyed in the production process.

You can find mezereum extract in bio-stores, or you can prepare your own ointment at home and apply it once each week to prevent pimples or other skin problems.

Conclusion

There are several ways to keep yourself healthy without paying large amounts of money for doctors every year. Throw away your collection of pills, and to start to pay attention to your inner self. You may still get sick every once in a while, and you may need to take a treatment. Howeverthese treatmentscan be natural and in complete harmony with your body.

It is more important to prevent a disease rather than focus on the treatment. A healthy lifestyle is the key to a happy life. All of the stressfulthoughts that you keep in your mind need to disappear. The most important goal to set for yourself is to be happy, to absorb positive energy from everything around you, and to learn to stop for a second and admire the world. Only in this way you will have a healthy spirit that will teach you how to bring peace into your life. No matter what kind of naturopathic treatment you decide to choose, make sure you put all of your positive energy into it, and soon enough, you will notice your life getting better and better.

ALL RIGHTS RESERVED. No part of this publication may be reproduced or transmitted in any form whatsoever, electronic, or mechanical, including photocopying, recording, or by any informational storage or retrieval system without express written, dated and signed permission from the author.

DISCLAIMER AND/OR LEGAL NOTICES:
Every effort has been made to accurately represent this book and it's potential. Results vary with every individual, and your results may or may not be different from those depicted. No promises, guarantees or warranties, whether stated or implied, have been made that you will produce any specific result from this book. Your efforts are individual and unique, and may vary from those shown. Your success depends on your efforts, background and motivation.

The material in this publication is provided for educational and informational purposes only and is not intended as medical advice. The information contained in this book should not be used to diagnose or treat any illness, metabolic disorder, disease or health problem. Always consult your physician or health care provider before beginning any nutrition or exercise program. Use of the programs, advice, and information contained in this book is at the sole choice and risk of the reader.